PRE-DIABETIC COOKBOOKS MEAL PLANS

PLANS

Delicious Recipes for a Healthy Lifestyle

T. John

COPYRIGHT PAGE

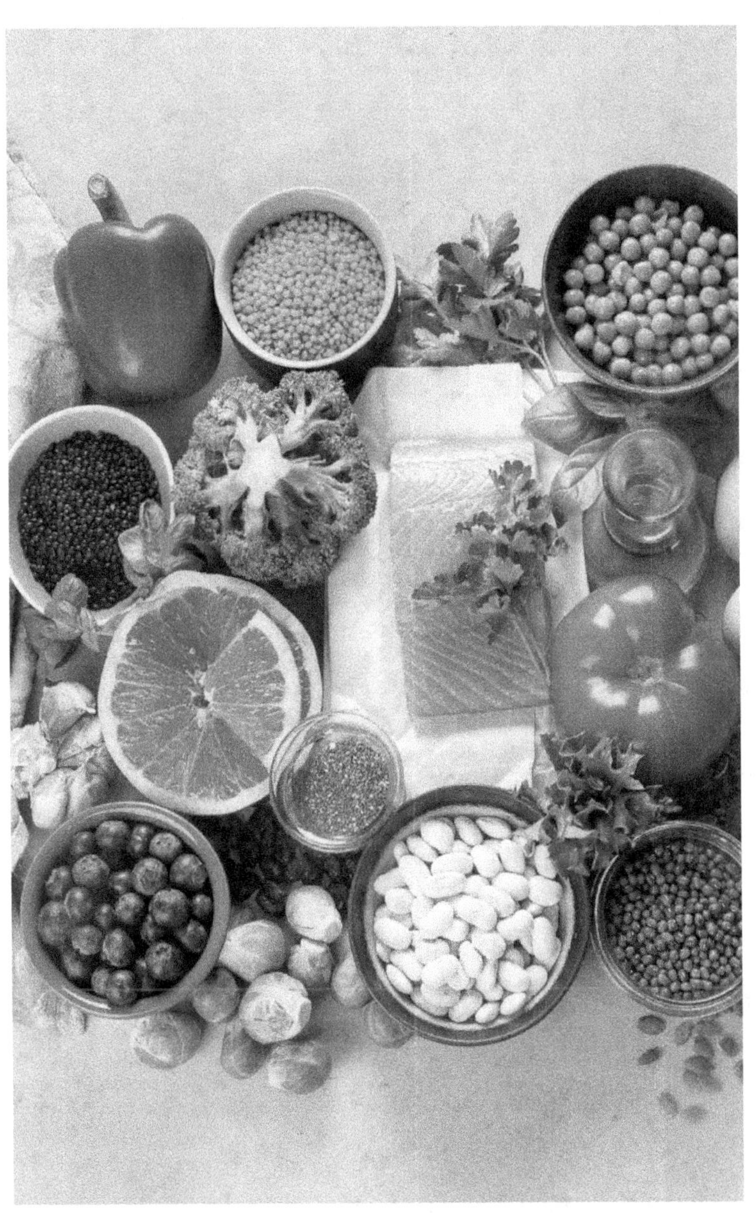

TABLE OF CONTENTS

Chapter 3: Lunch Recipes.. 43

Chapter 4: Dinner Recipes 62

Chapter 5: Snacks and Appetizers 84

INTRODUCTION

Pre-diabetes sits at a critical juncture, a silent warning before the possible onset of type 2 diabetes. Defined by blood sugar levels higher than normal but not high enough to be classified as diabetes, it represents a crucial window for intervention. While pre-diabetes may not have noticeable symptoms, its consequences can be significant, increasing the risk of heart disease, stroke, and other serious health conditions.

Fortunately, the path forward from pre-diabetes is paved with positive action. Diet serves as a powerful tool in this journey, offering a way to manage blood sugar levels and lower the risk of developing diabetes. Understanding the role of food in pre-diabetes management is essential for taking control of your health and embracing a future of well-being.

Diet: The Bedrock of Pre-diabetes Management

Nourishing your body with the right foods is the cornerstone of managing pre-diabetes. By making informed choices about what you eat, you can directly influence your blood sugar levels and promote overall health.

Here's how diet impacts pre-diabetes:

Carbohydrates: The type and quantity of carbohydrates you consume significantly impact your blood sugar. Refined carbohydrates, like white bread and sugary drinks, cause rapid blood sugar spikes. Opting for whole grains, fruits, and vegetables instead provides sustained energy and helps regulate blood sugar.

Fiber: This dietary hero plays a crucial role in digestion and blood sugar control. Fiber slows down the absorption of carbohydrates, preventing blood sugar spikes. Aim for 25-35 grams of fiber daily from whole grains, fruits, vegetables, and legumes.

Healthy Fats: Contrary to popular belief, incorporating healthy fats into your diet is beneficial. Choose unsaturated fats found in avocados, nuts, seeds, and olive oil. These fats promote satiety, improve insulin sensitivity, and reduce inflammation.

Protein: Lean protein sources like fish, poultry, beans, and lentils help stabilize blood sugar levels and keep you feeling full longer. They also contribute to building and maintaining muscle mass, which further aids in blood sugar control.

Sugar: Excess sugar intake is a major contributor to pre-diabetes and diabetes. Limit added sugars found in processed foods, sugary drinks, and sweets. Opt for naturally occurring sugars from fruits in moderation.

Navigating the Pre-diabetes Meal Plan

While general dietary guidelines are important, creating a personalized meal plan tailored to your needs and preferences is crucial for long-term success. Working with a registered dietitian or healthcare professional can help you develop a plan that fits your lifestyle and dietary requirements.

Here are some key strategies for crafting a pre-diabetes meal plan:

- **Focus on whole foods**: Prioritize unprocessed, whole foods like fruits, vegetables, whole grains, lean protein sources, and healthy fats.
- **Plan balanced meals and snacks**: Aim for meals and snacks that include a variety of food groups: carbohydrates, protein, healthy fats, and non-starchy vegetables. This helps ensure you receive essential nutrients while managing blood sugar levels.
- **Moderate portion sizes**: Pay attention to portion sizes to prevent overeating and subsequent blood sugar spikes. Utilize tools like the plate method, which encourages filling half your plate with non-starchy vegetables, a quarter with lean protein, and a quarter with whole grains.

- **Choose cooking methods wisely**: Opt for healthy cooking methods like grilling, baking, steaming, and boiling to preserve nutrients and minimize added fats.

- **Read food labels carefully**: Pay close attention to serving sizes, carbohydrate content, and added sugar content while making food choices.

- **Make gradual changes**: Don't try to overhaul your diet overnight. Introduce changes gradually to build sustainable healthy eating habits.

- Stay hydrated: Drinking plenty of water throughout the day helps regulate blood sugar and keep you feeling full.

Additional Tips for Optimal Pre-diabetes Management:

- **Regular physical activity**: Combine healthy eating with regular physical activity, aiming for at least 150 minutes of moderate-intensity exercise per week.

- **Stress management**: Chronic stress can worsen blood sugar control. Practice stress management techniques like yoga, meditation, or deep breathing.

- **Regular checkups**: Maintain regular communication with your healthcare provider to monitor your blood sugar levels and progress.

By understanding the role of diet in pre-diabetes management and adopting a personalized meal plan, you can significantly improve your health and well-being. Remember, it's not about deprivation but about making informed, positive choices that empower you to take control of your health and embrace a future free from diabetes.

Chapter 1: 30 Day Meal Plan

Week 1:

Day 1:

- Breakfast: Quinoa Breakfast Bowl
- Lunch: Grilled Chicken Salad with Avocado
- Dinner: Baked Salmon with Lemon and Dill
- Snack: Guacamole with Veggie Sticks
- Dessert: Berry and Greek Yogurt Popsicles

Day 2:

- Breakfast: Greek Yogurt Parfait
- Lunch: Quinoa and Black Bean Bowl
- Dinner: Quinoa-Stuffed Acorn Squash
- Snack: Hummus and Whole Wheat Pita
- Dessert: Dark Chocolate-Dipped Strawberries

Day 3:

- Breakfast: Veggie Omelette
- Lunch: Turkey and Vegetable Wrap
- Dinner: Grilled Vegetable Skewers with Chicken

- Snack: Greek Yogurt Dip with Cucumber Slices
- Dessert: Baked Apples with Cinnamon

Day 4:

- Breakfast: Chia Seed Pudding
- Lunch: Lentil and Vegetable Soup
- Dinner: Turkey and Sweet Potato Hash
- Snack: Roasted Chickpeas
- Dessert: Almond Flour Banana Bread

Day 5:

- Breakfast: Avocado Toast with Poached Egg
- Lunch: Salmon and Asparagus Foil Pack
- Dinner: Spaghetti Squash with Tomato and Basil Sauce
- Snack: Sliced Apple with Almond Butter
- Dessert: Chia Seed Chocolate Pudding

Day 6:

- Breakfast: Spinach and Feta Frittata
- Lunch: Chickpea and Vegetable Stir-Fry
- Dinner: Cauliflower and Broccoli Casserole

- Snack: Caprese Skewers
- Dessert: Coconut and Berry Parfait

Day 7:

- Breakfast: Berry Smoothie Bowl
- Lunch: Mediterranean Quinoa Salad
- Dinner: Cod with Garlic and Herb Butter
- Snack: Edamame with Sea Salt
- Dessert: Mango Sorbet

Week 2:

Day 8:

- Breakfast: Whole Grain Pancakes with Berries
- Lunch: Turkey and Quinoa Stuffed Peppers
- Dinner: Eggplant and Chickpea Curry
- Snack: Trail Mix with Nuts and Dried Fruits
- Dessert: Pumpkin Pie Smoothie

Day 9:

- Breakfast: Almond and Berry Breakfast Muffins
- Lunch: Zucchini Noodles with Pesto and Cherry Tomatoes

- Dinner: Baked Chicken Breast with Rosemary

- Snack: Cottage Cheese with Pineapple

- Dessert: Oatmeal Raisin Cookies

Day 10:

- Breakfast: Sweet Potato Hash with Turkey Sausage

- Lunch: Sweet Potato and Black Bean Quesadilla

- Dinner: Stir-Fried Tofu with Vegetables

- Snack: Stuffed Grape Leaves

- Dessert: Greek Yogurt Cheesecake Bites

Day 11:

- Breakfast: Green Smoothie with Kale and Pineapple

- Lunch: Shrimp and Broccoli Stir-Fry

- Dinner: Butternut Squash and Kale Risotto

- Snack: Veggie Spring Rolls with Peanut Sauce

- Dessert: Lemon Poppy Seed Muffins

Day 12:

- Breakfast: Oatmeal with Nuts and Berries

- Lunch: Spinach and Mushroom Quiche

- Dinner: Beef and Vegetable Skillet

- Snack: Baked Sweet Potato Fries
- Dessert: Mixed Berry Crisp

Day 13:

- Breakfast: Breakfast Burrito with Black Beans
- Lunch: Greek Chicken Wrap
- Dinner: Stuffed Bell Peppers with Quinoa and Black Beans
- Snack: Cheese and Whole Grain Crackers
- Dessert: Avocado Chocolate Mousse

Day 14:

- Breakfast: Cottage Cheese and Fruit Bowl
- Lunch: Cauliflower Fried Rice
- Dinner: Shrimp and Zucchini Noodles
- Snack: Antipasto Platter with Olives and Cheese
- Dessert: Peach and Almond Crumble

Week 3:

Day 15:

- Breakfast: Tomato and Basil Breakfast Sandwich
- Lunch: Caprese Salad with Balsamic Glaze

- Dinner: Teriyaki Salmon with Steamed Broccoli
- Snack: Cucumber Roll-Ups with Turkey and Cream Cheese
- Dessert: Raspberry and Almond Energy Bites

Day 16:

- Breakfast: Quinoa Breakfast Bowl
- Lunch: Grilled Chicken Salad with Avocado
- Dinner: Baked Salmon with Lemon and Dill
- Snack: Guacamole with Veggie Sticks
- Dessert: Berry and Greek Yogurt Popsicles

Day 17:

- Breakfast: Greek Yogurt Parfait
- Lunch: Quinoa and Black Bean Bowl
- Dinner: Quinoa-Stuffed Acorn Squash
- Snack: Hummus and Whole Wheat Pita
- Dessert: Dark Chocolate-Dipped Strawberries

Day 18:

- Breakfast: Veggie Omelette
- Lunch: Turkey and Vegetable Wrap

- Dinner: Grilled Vegetable Skewers with Chicken
- Snack: Greek Yogurt Dip with Cucumber Slices
- Dessert: Baked Apples with Cinnamon

Day 19:

- Breakfast: Chia Seed Pudding
- Lunch: Lentil and Vegetable Soup
- Dinner: Turkey and Sweet Potato Hash
- Snack: Roasted Chickpeas
- Dessert: Almond Flour Banana Bread

Day 20:

- Breakfast: Avocado Toast with Poached Egg
- Lunch: Salmon and Asparagus Foil Pack
- Dinner: Spaghetti Squash with Tomato and Basil Sauce
- Snack: Sliced Apple with Almond Butter
- Dessert: Chia Seed Chocolate Pudding

Day 21:

- Breakfast: Spinach and Feta Frittata
- Lunch: Chickpea and Vegetable Stir-Fry

- Dinner: Cauliflower and Broccoli Casserole
- Snack: Caprese Skewers
- Dessert: Coconut and Berry Parfait

Week 4:

Day 22:

- Breakfast: Whole Grain Pancakes with Berries
- Lunch: Turkey and Quinoa Stuffed Peppers
- Dinner: Eggplant and Chickpea Curry
- Snack: Trail Mix with Nuts and Dried Fruits
- Dessert: Pumpkin Pie Smoothie

Day 23:

- Breakfast: Almond and Berry Breakfast Muffins
- Lunch: Zucchini Noodles with Pesto and Cherry Tomatoes
- Dinner: Baked Chicken Breast with Rosemary
- Snack: Cottage Cheese with Pineapple
- Dessert: Oatmeal Raisin Cookies

Day 24:

- Breakfast: Sweet Potato Hash with Turkey Sausage

- Lunch: Sweet Potato and Black Bean Quesadilla
- Dinner: Stir-Fried Tofu with Vegetables
- Snack: Stuffed Grape Leaves
- Dessert: Greek Yogurt Cheesecake Bites

Day 25:

- Breakfast: Green Smoothie with Kale and Pineapple
- Lunch: Shrimp and Broccoli Stir-Fry
- Dinner: Butternut Squash and Kale Risotto
- Snack: Veggie Spring Rolls with Peanut Sauce
- Dessert: Lemon Poppy Seed Muffins

Day 26:

- Breakfast: Oatmeal with Nuts and Berries
- Lunch: Spinach and Mushroom Quiche
- Dinner: Beef and Vegetable Skillet
- Snack: Baked Sweet Potato Fries
- Dessert: Mixed Berry Crisp

Day 27:

- Breakfast: Breakfast Burrito with Black Beans
- Lunch: Greek Chicken Wrap

- Dinner: Stuffed Bell Peppers with Quinoa and Black Beans
- Snack: Cheese and Whole Grain Crackers
- Dessert: Avocado Chocolate Mousse

Day 28:

- Breakfast: Cottage Cheese and Fruit Bowl
- Lunch: Cauliflower Fried Rice
- Dinner: Shrimp and Zucchini Noodles
- Snack: Antipasto Platter with Olives and Cheese
- Dessert: Peach and Almond Crumble

Day 29:

- Breakfast: Tomato and Basil Breakfast Sandwich
- Lunch: Caprese Salad with Balsamic Glaze
- Dinner: Teriyaki Salmon with Steamed Broccoli
- Snack: Cucumber Roll-Ups with Turkey and Cream Cheese
- Dessert: Raspberry and Almond Energy Bites

Day 30:

- Breakfast: Quinoa Breakfast Bowl

- Lunch: Grilled Chicken Salad with Avocado

- Dinner: Baked Salmon with Lemon and Dill

- Snack: Guacamole with Veggie Sticks

- Dessert: Berry and Greek Yogurt Popsicles

Feel free to adjust the plan based on your preferences and dietary needs. Congratulations on completing the 30-day prediabetic meal plan!

Chapter 2: Breakfast Recipes

In this chapter, we present a delightful array of breakfast recipes tailored for those seeking a balanced start, especially those managing prediabetes. Each recipe is crafted with wholesome ingredients, ensuring not only a delicious meal but also one that supports your health goals.

Quinoa Breakfast Bowl

Ingredients:

- 1/2 cup quinoa
- 1 cup almond milk
- 1 tablespoon honey
- 1/4 cup chopped nuts (almonds, walnuts)
- 1/2 cup mixed berries (strawberries, blueberries)

Instructions:

1. Rinse quinoa thoroughly and cook it in almond milk until it simmers.
2. Stir in honey and let it simmer until quinoa is cooked.
3. Top with chopped nuts and mixed berries.

4. Enjoy this protein-packed bowl!

Nutrition Information:

- Calories: 350
- Protein: 12g
- Carbohydrates: 55g
- Fat: 10g
- Fiber: 8g
- Sugar: 10g
- Portion Size: 1 bowl

Greek Yogurt Parfait

Ingredients:

- 1 cup Greek yogurt
- 1/2 cup granola
- 1/4 cup honey
- 1/2 cup mixed fruits (kiwi, mango)

Instructions:

1. Layer Greek yogurt, granola, and mixed fruits in a glass.
2. Drizzle honey between layers.

3. Repeat for a visually appealing and tasty parfait.

Nutrition Information:

- Calories: 300
- Protein: 15g
- Carbohydrates: 45g
- Fat: 8g
- Fiber: 6g
- Sugar: 20g
- Portion Size: 1 parfait

Veggie Omelette

Ingredients:

- 2 eggs
- 1/4 cup bell peppers (mixed colors), diced
- 1/4 cup cherry tomatoes, halved
- 1/4 cup spinach, chopped
- 1/4 cup feta cheese, crumbled

Instructions:

1. Whisk eggs and pour into a heated, oiled pan.

2. Sprinkle bell peppers, cherry tomatoes, spinach, and feta on one side.

3. Fold the omelette in half and cook until eggs are set.

4. Serve with a side of fresh herbs.

Nutrition Information:

- Calories: 250
- Protein: 18g
- Carbohydrates: 8g
- Fat: 15g
- Fiber: 2g
- Sugar: 3g
- Portion Size: 1 omelette

Chia Seed Pudding

Ingredients:

- 2 tablespoons chia seeds
- 1 cup almond milk
- 1/2 teaspoon vanilla extract
- 1 tablespoon maple syrup
- Fresh berries for topping

Instructions:

1. Mix chia seeds, almond milk, vanilla extract, and maple syrup in a jar.
2. Stir well and refrigerate overnight.
3. Top with fresh berries before serving.

Nutrition Information:

- Calories: 180
- Protein: 5g
- Carbohydrates: 25g
- Fat: 8g
- Fiber: 10g
- Sugar: 10g
- Portion Size: 1 serving

Avocado Toast with Poached Egg

Ingredients:

- 1 slice whole-grain bread
- 1/2 ripe avocado, mashed
- 1 poached egg
- Salt and pepper to taste
- Red pepper flakes (optional)

Instructions:

1. Toast the bread until golden brown.

2. Spread mashed avocado on the toast.

3. Top with a poached egg and season with salt, pepper,
    and red pepper flakes if desired.

Nutrition Information:

- Calories: 220

- Protein: 10g

- Carbohydrates: 18g

- Fat: 14g

- Fiber: 7g

- Sugar: 1g

- Portion Size: 1 serving

Spinach and Feta Frittata

Ingredients:

- 4 eggs

- 1 cup fresh spinach, chopped

- 1/4 cup feta cheese, crumbled

- 1/4 cup red bell pepper, diced

- Salt and pepper to taste

Instructions:

1. Preheat the oven to 350°F (175°C).

2. Whisk eggs and mix in spinach, feta, and red bell pepper.

3. Pour the mixture into a greased baking dish and bake until set.

4. Slice and serve with a sprinkle of salt and pepper.

Nutrition Information:

- Calories: 280
- Protein: 18g
- Carbohydrates: 4g
- Fat: 20g
- Fiber: 2g
- Sugar: 1g
- Portion Size: 1 slice

Berry Smoothie Bowl

Ingredients:

- 1 cup mixed berries (strawberries, blueberries, raspberries)
- 1/2 banana, sliced

- 1/2 cup Greek yogurt

- 1/4 cup granola

- 1 tablespoon honey

Instructions:

1. Blend mixed berries, banana, and Greek yogurt until smooth.

2. Pour into a bowl and top with granola and a drizzle of honey.

Nutrition Information:

- Calories: 300

- Protein: 15g

- Carbohydrates: 50g

- Fat: 5g

- Fiber: 8g

- Sugar: 25g

- Portion Size: 1 bowl

Whole Grain Pancakes with Berries

Ingredients:

- 1 cup whole wheat flour

- 1 tablespoon baking powder
- 1 egg
- 1 cup almond milk
- 1 cup mixed berries for topping

Instructions:

1. Mix whole wheat flour and baking powder in a bowl.
2. Add egg and almond milk, stirring until smooth.
3. Pour batter onto a hot griddle to make pancakes.
4. Top with mixed berries before serving.

Nutrition Information:

- Calories: 280
- Protein: 10g
- Carbohydrates: 45g
- Fat: 8g
- Fiber: 7g
- Sugar: 8g
- Portion Size: 2 pancakes

Almond and Berry Breakfast Muffins

Ingredients:

- 1 cup almond flour
- 1/2 cup oats
- 1 teaspoon baking powder
- 2 eggs
- 1/4 cup almond milk
- 1/2 cup mixed berries

Instructions:

1. Preheat the oven to 350°F (175°C) and line a muffin tin with liners.
2. In a bowl, combine almond flour, oats, and baking powder.
3. In another bowl, whisk eggs and mix in almond milk.
4. Combine wet and dry ingredients, then fold in mixed berries.
5. Spoon the batter into muffin cups and bake until golden.

Nutrition Information:

- Calories: 220

- Protein: 9g
- Carbohydrates: 15g
- Fat: 15g
- Fiber: 4g
- Sugar: 4g
- Portion Size: 1 muffin

Sweet Potato Hash with Turkey Sausage

Ingredients:

- 1 sweet potato, grated
- 1/2 lb turkey sausage, crumbled
- 1/2 onion, diced
- 1 bell pepper, diced
- 1 tablespoon olive oil

Instructions:

1. Heat olive oil in a skillet and sauté onion and bell pepper.
2. Add turkey sausage and cook until browned.
3. Stir in grated sweet potato and cook until tender.

Nutrition Information:

- Calories: 280
- Protein: 15g
- Carbohydrates: 25g
- Fat: 14g
- Fiber: 5g
- Sugar: 8g
- Portion Size: 1 serving

Green Smoothie with Kale and Pineapple

Ingredients:

- 1 cup kale, stems removed
- 1/2 cup pineapple chunks
- 1/2 banana
- 1/2 cup Greek yogurt
- 1/2 cup coconut water

Instructions:

1. Blend kale, pineapple, banana, Greek yogurt, and coconut water until smooth.

2. Pour into a glass and enjoy this refreshing green smoothie.

Nutrition Information:

- Calories: 200
- Protein: 10g
- Carbohydrates: 40g
- Fat: 2g
- Fiber: 6g
- Sugar: 20g
- Portion Size: 1 smoothie

Oatmeal with Nuts and Berries

Ingredients:

- 1/2 cup rolled oats
- 1 cup almond milk
- 1/4 cup mixed nuts (walnuts, almonds)
- 1/2 cup mixed berries
- 1 tablespoon honey

Instructions:

1. Cook rolled oats in almond milk until creamy.

2. Top with mixed nuts, berries, and a drizzle of honey.

Nutrition Information:

- Calories: 300
- Protein: 10g
- Carbohydrates: 40g
- Fat: 12g
- Fiber: 8g
- Sugar: 12g
- Portion Size: 1 serving

Breakfast Burrito with Black Beans

Ingredients:

- 2 whole wheat tortillas
- 2 eggs, scrambled
- 1/2 cup black beans, cooked
- 1/4 cup salsa
- 1/4 cup shredded cheese

Instructions:

1. Scramble eggs and set aside.

2. Warm tortillas and assemble with scrambled eggs, black beans, salsa, and shredded cheese.

3. Roll into a burrito and enjoy a savory breakfast.

Nutrition Information:

- Calories: 320
- Protein: 18g
- Carbohydrates: 35g
- Fat: 12g
- Fiber: 8g
- Sugar: 3g
- Portion Size: 1 burrito

Cottage Cheese and Fruit Bowl

Ingredients:

- 1 cup low-fat cottage cheese
- 1/2 cup pineapple chunks
- 1/2 cup mango chunks
- 1/4 cup chopped nuts (cashews, almonds)

Instructions:

1. Combine cottage cheese, pineapple, mango, and chopped nuts in a bowl.
2. Mix well and savor the sweet and savory flavors.

Nutrition Information:

- Calories: 250
- Protein: 20g
- Carbohydrates: 30g
- Fat: 8g
- Fiber: 4g
- Sugar: 20g
- Portion Size: 1 bowl

Tomato and Basil Breakfast Sandwich

Ingredients:

- 1 whole grain English muffin
- 1 egg, fried
- 1 slice tomato
- Fresh basil leaves

- Salt and pepper to taste

Instructions:

1. Toast the English muffin and fry the egg to your liking.
2. Assemble the sandwich with the fried egg, tomato slice, fresh basil, and season with salt and pepper.

Nutrition Information:

- Calories: 230
- Protein: 12g
- Carbohydrates: 30g
- Fat: 8g
- Fiber: 6g
- Sugar: 3g
- Portion Size: 1 sandwich

Chapter 3: Lunch Recipes

Welcome to Chapter 3 of our Prediabetes Cookbooks Meal Plans, where we explore a delightful array of Lunch Recipes designed to nourish your body while keeping blood sugar levels in check. These recipes are not only delicious but also crafted with a focus on balance and nutritional value.

Grilled Chicken Salad with Avocado:

Ingredients:

- 2 boneless, skinless chicken breasts
- 1 avocado, sliced
- Mixed salad greens
- Cherry tomatoes, halved
- Red onion, thinly sliced
- Balsamic vinaigrette dressing

Instructions:

1. Season chicken breasts with salt and pepper.
2. Grill until fully cooked, then slice.

3. In a large bowl, combine salad greens, cherry tomatoes, red onion, and sliced avocado.

4. Top with grilled chicken slices.

5. Drizzle with balsamic vinaigrette.

Nutrition Information:

- Calories: 350
- Protein: 25g
- Carbohydrates: 15g
- Fat: 20g
- Fiber: 8g
- Sugar: 5g
- Portion Size: 1 serving

Quinoa and Black Bean Bowl:

Ingredients:

- 1 cup cooked quinoa
- 1 cup black beans, drained and rinsed
- Corn kernels
- Red bell pepper, diced
- Avocado, diced
- Lime juice

- Cilantro, chopped

Instructions:

1. In a bowl, combine quinoa, black beans, corn, and diced red bell pepper.
2. Add diced avocado.
3. Squeeze lime juice over the mixture.
4. Sprinkle with chopped cilantro.

Nutrition Information:

- Calories: 300
- Protein: 12g
- Carbohydrates: 45g
- Fat: 10g
- Fiber: 12g
- Sugar: 2g
- Portion Size: 1 serving

Turkey and Vegetable Wrap:

Ingredients:

- Whole-grain tortilla
- Lean ground turkey

- Bell peppers, thinly sliced
- Spinach leaves
- Hummus
- Feta cheese, crumbled

Instructions:

1. Cook ground turkey until browned.
2. Warm the tortilla and spread hummus over it.
3. Layer with cooked turkey, bell peppers, spinach, and crumbled feta.
4. Roll tightly into a wrap.

Nutrition Information:

- Calories: 320
- Protein: 22g
- Carbohydrates: 25g
- Fat: 15g
- Fiber: 6g
- Sugar: 3g
- Portion Size: 1 serving

Lentil and Vegetable Soup:

Ingredients:

- 1 cup lentils, rinsed
- Carrots, chopped
- Celery, chopped
- Onion, diced
- Garlic, minced
- Vegetable broth
- Spinach leaves
- Italian seasoning

Instructions:

1. Combine lentils, carrots, celery, onion, and garlic in a pot with vegetable broth.
2. Simmer until lentils are tender.
3. Stir in spinach leaves and Italian seasoning.
4. Cook until spinach wilts.

Nutrition Information:

- Calories: 250
- Protein: 18g
- Carbohydrates: 40g

- Fat: 2g

- Fiber: 15g

- Sugar: 5g

- Portion Size: 1 serving

Salmon and Asparagus Foil Pack:

Ingredients:

- Salmon fillet

- Asparagus spears

- Lemon slices

- Garlic, minced

- Olive oil

- Fresh dill

Instructions:

1. Place salmon on a piece of foil.

2. Arrange asparagus around the salmon.

3. Top with lemon slices and minced garlic.

4. Drizzle with olive oil and sprinkle fresh dill.

5. Seal the foil and bake until salmon is cooked.

Nutrition Information:

- Calories: 280
- Protein: 30g
- Carbohydrates: 8g
- Fat: 15g
- Fiber: 3g
- Sugar: 2g
- Portion Size: 1 serving

Chickpea and Vegetable Stir-Fry:

Ingredients:

- Chickpeas, drained and rinsed
- Broccoli florets
- Bell peppers, sliced
- Snow peas
- Soy sauce
- Ginger, grated
- Garlic, minced

Instructions:

1. Stir-fry chickpeas, broccoli, bell peppers, and snow peas in a pan.

2. Add soy sauce, grated ginger, and minced garlic.

3. Cook until vegetables are tender-crisp.

Nutrition Information:

- Calories: 220

- Protein: 12g

- Carbohydrates: 35g

- Fat: 5g

- Fiber: 9g

- Sugar: 7g

- Portion Size: 1 serving

Mediterranean Quinoa Salad:

Ingredients:

- Cooked quinoa

- Cherry tomatoes, halved

- Cucumber, diced

- Kalamata olives, sliced

- Red onion, finely chopped

- Feta cheese, crumbled

- Olive oil and lemon dressing

Instructions:

1. In a large bowl, combine quinoa, cherry tomatoes, cucumber, olives, red onion, and feta.
2. Drizzle with olive oil and lemon dressing.
3. Toss gently to combine.

Nutrition Information:

- Calories: 290
- Protein: 10g
- Carbohydrates: 30g
- Fat: 15g
- Fiber: 5g
- Sugar: 3g
- Portion Size: 1 serving

Turkey and Quinoa Stuffed Peppers:

Ingredients:

- Bell peppers, halved
- Lean ground turkey
- Quinoa, cooked
- Black beans, drained and rinsed
- Corn kernels

- Tomato sauce

- Mexican seasoning

Instructions:

1. Preheat the oven and cook ground turkey.

2. Mix turkey with cooked quinoa, black beans, corn, and tomato sauce.

3. Stuff bell peppers with the mixture.

4. Bake until peppers are tender.

Nutrition Information:

- Calories: 340

- Protein: 25g

- Carbohydrates: 35g

- Fat: 12g

- Fiber: 8g

- Sugar: 5g

- Portion Size: 1 serving

Zucchini Noodles with Pesto and Cherry Tomatoes:

Ingredients:

- Zucchini, spiralized into noodles
- Cherry tomatoes, halved
- Pesto sauce
- Parmesan cheese, grated
- Pine nuts

Instructions:

1. Spiralize zucchini into noodle shapes.
2. Toss zucchini noodles with pesto, cherry tomatoes, and Parmesan cheese.
3. Toast pine nuts and sprinkle on top.

Nutrition Information:

- Calories: 220
- Protein: 8g
- Carbohydrates: 15g
- Fat: 18g
- Fiber: 5g
- Sugar: 3g

- Portion Size: 1 serving

Sweet Potato and Black Bean Quesadilla:

Ingredients:

- Whole-grain tortilla
- Sweet potato, cooked and mashed
- Black beans, mashed
- Red onion, diced
- Cumin and chili powder
- Shredded cheese (cheddar or Mexican blend)

Instructions:

1. Spread mashed sweet potato on a tortilla.
2. Top with mashed black beans, diced red onion, and spices.
3. Sprinkle with shredded cheese and fold in half.
4. Cook until cheese is melted.

Nutrition Information:

- Calories: 280

- Protein: 12g
- Carbohydrates: 40g
- Fat: 8g
- Fiber: 10g
- Sugar: 5g
- Portion Size: 1 serving

Shrimp and Broccoli Stir-Fry:

Ingredients:

- Shrimp, peeled and deveined
- Broccoli florets
- Bell peppers, sliced
- Snow peas
- Soy sauce
- Garlic, minced
- Sesame oil

Instructions:

1. Stir-fry shrimp, broccoli, bell peppers, and snow peas in a pan.
2. Add minced garlic, soy sauce, and a drizzle of sesame oil.

3. Cook until shrimp is pink and vegetables are crisp-tender.

Nutrition Information:

- Calories: 250
- Protein: 20g
- Carbohydrates: 15g
- Fat: 10g
- Fiber: 5g
- Sugar: 3g
- Portion Size: 1 serving

Spinach and Mushroom Quiche:

Ingredients:

- Pie crust (whole-grain)
- Eggs
- Spinach, chopped
- Mushrooms, sliced
- Milk (or milk substitute)
- Swiss cheese, shredded
- Salt and pepper

Instructions:

1. Preheat the oven and bake the pie crust.

2. Whisk together eggs, milk, salt, and pepper.

3. Stir in chopped spinach, sliced mushrooms, and shredded Swiss cheese.

4. Pour the mixture into the baked crust and bake until set.

Nutrition Information:

- Calories: 280
- Protein: 15g
- Carbohydrates: 20g
- Fat: 15g
- Fiber: 3g
- Sugar: 2g
- Portion Size: 1 serving

Greek Chicken Wrap:

Ingredients:

- Grilled chicken breast, sliced
- Whole-grain wrap
- Tzatziki sauce

- Cherry tomatoes, halved

- Cucumber, thinly sliced

- Red onion, thinly sliced

- Feta cheese, crumbled

Instructions:

1. Lay out the whole-grain wrap.

2. Arrange sliced grilled chicken, tzatziki sauce, cherry tomatoes, cucumber, red onion, and crumbled feta.

3. Roll up the wrap and secure with toothpicks.

Nutrition Information:

- Calories: 320

- Protein: 25g

- Carbohydrates: 30g

- Fat: 12g

- Fiber: 5g

- Sugar: 4g

- Portion Size: 1 serving

Cauliflower Fried Rice:

Ingredients:

- Cauliflower, grated
- Shrimp, cooked and chopped
- Peas and carrots, diced
- Scallions, sliced
- Eggs, beaten
- Soy sauce
- Sesame oil

Instructions:

1. Stir-fry grated cauliflower, cooked shrimp, peas, carrots, and sliced scallions in a pan.
2. Push the mixture to the side, pour beaten eggs into the pan, and scramble.
3. Mix everything together, add soy sauce and sesame oil, and stir-fry until heated through.

Nutrition Information:

- Calories: 230
- Protein: 20g
- Carbohydrates: 15g

- Fat: 10g

- Fiber: 6g

- Sugar: 4g

- Portion Size: 1 serving

Caprese Salad with Balsamic Glaze:

Ingredients:

- Tomatoes, sliced

- Fresh mozzarella, sliced

- Fresh basil leaves

- Balsamic glaze

- Olive oil

- Salt and pepper

Instructions:

1. Arrange alternating slices of tomatoes and fresh mozzarella on a serving platter.

2. Tuck fresh basil leaves between the slices.

3. Drizzle with balsamic glaze and olive oil.

4. Sprinkle with salt and pepper to taste.

Nutrition Information:

- Calories: 200
- Protein: 12g
- Carbohydrates: 10g
- Fat: 15g
- Fiber: 2g
- Sugar: 6g
- Portion Size: 1 serving

Chapter 4: Dinner Recipes

These recipes are crafted with a mindful selection of ingredients to promote balanced nutrition, keeping in mind the dietary needs of individuals managing prediabetes. Each recipe is designed to be not only flavorful but also supportive of a healthy lifestyle.

Baked Salmon with Lemon and Dill

Ingredients:

- 4 salmon fillets
- 2 tablespoons olive oil
- 1 lemon, sliced
- 2 tablespoons fresh dill, chopped
- Salt and pepper to taste

Instructions:

1. Preheat the oven to 375°F (190°C).
2. Place salmon fillets on a baking sheet.
3. Drizzle olive oil over the fillets and season with salt and pepper.

4. Lay lemon slices on top of the salmon and sprinkle with fresh dill.

5. Bake for 15-20 minutes or until salmon is cooked through.

6. Serve with a side of steamed broccoli.

Nutrition Information (per serving):

- Calories: 300

- Protein: 25g

- Carbohydrates: 2g

- Fat: 20g

- Fiber: 1g

- Sugar: 0g

- Portion Size: 1 fillet

Quinoa-Stuffed Acorn Squash

Ingredients:

- 2 acorn squashes, halved

- 1 cup quinoa, cooked

- 1 cup black beans, drained and rinsed

- 1 cup cherry tomatoes, halved

- 1/2 cup feta cheese, crumbled

- 2 tablespoons olive oil
- Salt and pepper to taste

Instructions:

1. Preheat the oven to 400°F (200°C).
2. Scoop out the seeds from acorn squashes and place them on a baking sheet.
3. In a bowl, mix cooked quinoa, black beans, cherry tomatoes, and feta cheese.
4. Stuff each squash half with the quinoa mixture.
5. Drizzle with olive oil, sprinkle with salt and pepper.
6. Bake for 25-30 minutes or until the squash is tender.
7. Serve with a side salad.

Nutrition Information (per serving):

- Calories: 350
- Protein: 12g
- Carbohydrates: 45g
- Fat: 15g
- Fiber: 10g
- Sugar: 2g
- Portion Size: 1 stuffed squash half

Grilled Vegetable Skewers with Chicken

Ingredients:

- 1 lb chicken breast, cut into cubes
- 2 zucchinis, sliced
- 1 bell pepper, cut into chunks
- 1 red onion, cut into wedges
- 1 cup cherry tomatoes
- 2 tablespoons olive oil
- 1 teaspoon Italian seasoning
- Salt and pepper to taste

Instructions:

1. Preheat the grill to medium-high heat.
2. Thread chicken and vegetables onto skewers.
3. In a bowl, mix olive oil, Italian seasoning, salt, and pepper.
4. Brush the skewers with the olive oil mixture.
5. Grill for 10-15 minutes, turning occasionally, until chicken is cooked.
6. Serve with quinoa or brown rice.

Nutrition Information (per serving):

- Calories: 280
- Protein: 30g
- Carbohydrates: 15g
- Fat: 12g
- Fiber: 4g
- Sugar: 6g
- Portion Size: 2 skewers

Turkey and Sweet Potato Hash

Ingredients:

- 1 lb ground turkey
- 2 sweet potatoes, peeled and diced
- 1 bell pepper, chopped
- 1 onion, diced
- 2 cloves garlic, minced
- 1 teaspoon paprika
- Salt and pepper to taste
- 2 tablespoons olive oil

Instructions:

1. Heat olive oil in a skillet over medium heat.

2. Add ground turkey and cook until browned.

3. Add sweet potatoes, bell pepper, onion, and garlic to the skillet.

4. Season with paprika, salt, and pepper.

5. Cook until sweet potatoes are tender, stirring occasionally.

6. Serve hot, garnished with fresh herbs if desired.

Nutrition Information (per serving):

- Calories: 320
- Protein: 22g
- Carbohydrates: 25g
- Fat: 15g
- Fiber: 5g
- Sugar: 6g
- Portion Size: 1 cup

Spaghetti Squash with Tomato and Basil Sauce

Ingredients:

- 1 spaghetti squash, halved

- 2 cups cherry tomatoes, halved

- 2 cloves garlic, minced

- 1/4 cup fresh basil, chopped

- 2 tablespoons olive oil

- Salt and pepper to taste

- Grated Parmesan cheese (optional)

Instructions:

1. Preheat the oven to 400°F (200°C).

2. Roast spaghetti squash halves, cut side down, for 40-45 minutes.

3. In a pan, sauté garlic in olive oil until fragrant.

4. Add cherry tomatoes and cook until softened.

5. Use a fork to scrape the spaghetti squash into "noodles."

6. Toss squash noodles with tomato and basil sauce.

7. Season with salt and pepper, and sprinkle with Parmesan if desired.

Nutrition Information (per serving):

- Calories: 220

- Protein: 5g

- Carbohydrates: 30g

- Fat: 10g

- Fiber: 6g

- Sugar: 12g

- Portion Size: 1 cup

Cauliflower and Broccoli Casserole

Ingredients:

- 1 head cauliflower, cut into florets

- 2 cups broccoli florets

- 1 cup cheddar cheese, shredded

- 1/2 cup Parmesan cheese, grated

- 1 cup Greek yogurt

- 2 cloves garlic, minced

- Salt and pepper to taste

Instructions:

1. Preheat the oven to 375°F (190°C).

2. Steam cauliflower and broccoli until slightly tender.

3. In a bowl, mix Greek yogurt, garlic, salt, and pepper.

4. Combine cauliflower and broccoli with the yogurt mixture.

5. Transfer to a baking dish, top with cheddar and Parmesan.

6. Bake for 20-25 minutes or until cheese is melted and bubbly.

Nutrition Information (per serving):

- Calories: 280

- Protein: 18g

- Carbohydrates: 15g

- Fat: 18g

- Fiber: 6g

- Sugar: 8g

- Portion Size: 1 cup

Cod with Garlic and Herb Butter

Ingredients:

- 4 cod fillets

- 4 tablespoons unsalted butter, melted

- 3 cloves garlic, minced

- 1 tablespoon fresh parsley, chopped

- 1 tablespoon fresh lemon juice

- Salt and pepper to taste

Instructions:

1. Preheat the oven to 400°F (200°C).

2. Place cod fillets on a baking sheet lined with parchment paper.

3. In a bowl, mix melted butter, minced garlic, parsley, lemon juice, salt, and pepper.

4. Brush the cod fillets with the butter mixture.

5. Bake for 12-15 minutes or until the fish flakes easily.

6. Serve with a side of steamed vegetables.

Nutrition Information (per serving):

- Calories: 220

- Protein: 25g

- Carbohydrates: 1g

- Fat: 13g

- Fiber: 0g

- Sugar: 0g

- Portion Size: 1 fillet

Eggplant and Chickpea Curry

Ingredients:

- 1 large eggplant, diced

- 1 can chickpeas, drained and rinsed
- 1 onion, finely chopped
- 2 cloves garlic, minced
- 1 can diced tomatoes
- 1 can coconut milk
- 2 tablespoons curry powder
- Salt and pepper to taste
- Fresh cilantro for garnish

Instructions:

1. In a pot, sauté onion and garlic until softened.
2. Add diced eggplant, chickpeas, diced tomatoes, and coconut milk.
3. Stir in curry powder, salt, and pepper.
4. Simmer for 20-25 minutes or until eggplant is tender.
5. Garnish with fresh cilantro before serving.
6. Serve over brown rice or quinoa.

Nutrition Information (per serving):

- Calories: 320
- Protein: 9g
- Carbohydrates: 40g

- Fat: 16g

- Fiber: 10g

- Sugar: 10g

- Portion Size: 1 cup

Baked Chicken Breast with Rosemary

Ingredients:

- 4 boneless, skinless chicken breasts

- 2 tablespoons olive oil

- 2 teaspoons fresh rosemary, chopped

- 1 teaspoon garlic powder

- Salt and pepper to taste

- Lemon wedges for serving

Instructions:

1. Preheat the oven to 400°F (200°C).

2. Place chicken breasts on a baking sheet.

3. Drizzle with olive oil and season with rosemary, garlic powder, salt, and pepper.

4. Bake for 25-30 minutes or until the chicken is cooked through.

5. Serve with lemon wedges for a burst of flavor.

Nutrition Information (per serving):

- Calories: 220

- Protein: 30g

- Carbohydrates: 1g

- Fat: 10g

- Fiber: 0g

- Sugar: 0g

- Portion Size: 1 chicken breast

Stir-Fried Tofu with Vegetables

Ingredients:

- 1 block firm tofu, pressed and cubed

- 2 cups broccoli florets

- 1 red bell pepper, sliced

- 1 carrot, julienned

- 3 tablespoons soy sauce

- 2 tablespoons sesame oil

- 1 tablespoon ginger, minced

- 2 cloves garlic, minced
- 1 tablespoon rice vinegar
- 1 tablespoon honey or maple syrup
- Sesame seeds for garnish

Instructions:

1. In a wok or skillet, heat sesame oil over medium-high heat.
2. Add cubed tofu and stir-fry until golden brown.
3. Add broccoli, bell pepper, and carrot to the tofu.
4. In a bowl, mix soy sauce, ginger, garlic, rice vinegar, and honey/maple syrup.
5. Pour the sauce over the tofu and vegetables, toss to coat evenly.
6. Stir-fry for an additional 3-5 minutes until vegetables are tender.
7. Garnish with sesame seeds before serving.

Nutrition Information (per serving):

- Calories: 280
- Protein: 18g
- Carbohydrates: 20g

- Fat: 15g

- Fiber: 6g

- Sugar: 8g

- Portion Size: 1 cup

Butternut Squash and Kale Risotto

Ingredients:

- 2 cups butternut squash, diced

- 1 cup Arborio rice

- 1 onion, finely chopped

- 2 cloves garlic, minced

- 4 cups vegetable broth, warm

- 1 cup kale, chopped

- 1/2 cup Parmesan cheese, grated

- 2 tablespoons olive oil

- Salt and pepper to taste

Instructions:

1. In a large pan, sauté onion and garlic in olive oil until translucent.

2. Add Arborio rice and cook for 1-2 minutes.

3. Pour in a ladle of warm vegetable broth, stirring constantly.

4. Continue adding broth gradually until rice is creamy and cooked.

5. Stir in butternut squash, kale, and Parmesan cheese.

6. Cook until squash is tender and kale is wilted.

7. Season with salt and pepper before serving.

Nutrition Information (per serving):

- Calories: 320
- Protein: 8g
- Carbohydrates: 60g
- Fat: 6g
- Fiber: 5g
- Sugar: 4g
- Portion Size: 1 cup

Beef and Vegetable Skillet

Ingredients:

- 1 lb lean ground beef
- 1 bell pepper, sliced
- 1 zucchini, sliced

- 1 onion, chopped
- 2 cloves garlic, minced
- 1 can diced tomatoes
- 1 tablespoon olive oil
- 1 teaspoon Italian seasoning
- Salt and pepper to taste

Instructions:

1. In a large skillet, brown ground beef in olive oil over medium heat.
2. Add onion and garlic, sauté until softened.
3. Stir in bell pepper and zucchini, cook until vegetables are tender.
4. Pour in diced tomatoes and sprinkle with Italian seasoning, salt, and pepper.
5. Simmer for 10-15 minutes until flavors meld.
6. Serve over quinoa or whole grain pasta.

Nutrition Information (per serving):

- Calories: 350
- Protein: 25g
- Carbohydrates: 20g

- Fat: 18g

- Fiber: 5g

- Sugar: 8g

- Portion Size: 1 cup

Stuffed Bell Peppers with Quinoa and Black Beans

Ingredients:

- 4 bell peppers, halved and seeds removed

- 1 cup quinoa, cooked

- 1 can black beans, drained and rinsed

- 1 cup corn kernels (fresh or frozen)

- 1 cup salsa

- 1 teaspoon cumin

- 1 teaspoon chili powder

- Salt and pepper to taste

- Shredded cheddar cheese for topping

Instructions:

1. Preheat the oven to 375°F (190°C).

2. In a bowl, combine cooked quinoa, black beans, corn, salsa, cumin, chili powder, salt, and pepper.

3. Stuff each bell pepper half with the quinoa mixture.

4. Place stuffed peppers in a baking dish, cover with foil.

5. Bake for 25-30 minutes until peppers are tender.

6. Remove foil, sprinkle with shredded cheddar, and bake until cheese melts.

Nutrition Information (per serving):

- Calories: 280
- Protein: 10g
- Carbohydrates: 50g
- Fat: 5g
- Fiber: 10g
- Sugar: 8g
- Portion Size: 2 pepper halves

Shrimp and Zucchini Noodles

Ingredients:

- 1 lb shrimp, peeled and deveined
- 4 medium zucchinis, spiralized into noodles

- 2 tablespoons olive oil

- 3 cloves garlic, minced

- 1 teaspoon red pepper flakes

- Juice of 1 lemon

- Salt and pepper to taste

- Fresh parsley for garnish

Instructions:

1. In a large pan, heat olive oil over medium heat.

2. Add shrimp and garlic, sauté until shrimp turn pink.

3. Add zucchini noodles, red pepper flakes, lemon juice, salt, and pepper.

4. Cook for 2-3 minutes until zucchini noodles are tender.

5. Garnish with fresh parsley before serving.

Nutrition Information (per serving):

- Calories: 220

- Protein: 25g

- Carbohydrates: 10g

- Fat: 10g

- Fiber: 3g

- Sugar: 5g
- Portion Size: 1.5 cups

Teriyaki Salmon with Steamed Broccoli

Ingredients:

- 4 salmon fillets
- 1/4 cup low-sodium soy sauce
- 2 tablespoons honey
- 1 tablespoon rice vinegar
- 1 teaspoon sesame oil
- 2 cloves garlic, minced
- 1 teaspoon ginger, grated
- 2 cups broccoli florets
- Sesame seeds for garnish

Instructions:

1. In a bowl, mix soy sauce, honey, rice vinegar, sesame oil, garlic, and ginger to make the teriyaki sauce.
2. Marinate salmon fillets in the sauce for 30 minutes.
3. Preheat the oven to 400°F (200°C).

4. Place marinated salmon on a baking sheet.

5. Bake for 15-20 minutes until salmon is cooked through.

6. Steam broccoli separately.

7. Serve salmon over a bed of steamed broccoli, garnish with sesame seeds.

Nutrition Information (per serving):

- Calories: 320

- Protein: 30g

- Carbohydrates: 15g

- Fat: 15g

- Fiber: 3g

- Sugar: 10g

- Portion Size: 1 fillet with broccoli

Chapter 5: Snacks and Appetizers

These tasty bites not only satisfy your cravings but also adhere to the principles of a balanced diet, keeping your prediabetes in check. From wholesome guacamole to inventive cucumber roll-ups, each recipe brings together vibrant flavors and nutritional goodness.

Guacamole with Veggie Sticks

Ingredients:

- 2 ripe avocados
- 1 small onion, finely diced
- 1 medium tomato, diced
- 1 clove garlic, minced
- 1 lime, juiced
- Salt and pepper to taste
- Assorted veggie sticks (carrots, bell peppers, cucumber)

Instructions:

1. In a bowl, mash the avocados.

2. Add the diced onion, tomato, minced garlic, and lime juice. Mix well.

3. Season with salt and pepper to taste.

4. Serve with an assortment of veggie sticks.

Nutrition Information (per serving):

- Calories: 120
- Protein: 2g
- Carbohydrates: 8g
- Fat: 10g
- Fiber: 5g
- Sugar: 1g
- Portion Size: 1/2 cup guacamole with veggie sticks

Hummus and Whole Wheat Pita

Ingredients:

- 1 can chickpeas, drained and rinsed
- 2 cloves garlic
- 1/4 cup tahini
- 2 tablespoons olive oil
- 1 lemon, juiced
- Salt to taste

- Whole wheat pita, cut into triangles

Instructions:

1. In a food processor, combine chickpeas, garlic, tahini, olive oil, and lemon juice.
2. Blend until smooth, adding water if needed for desired consistency.
3. Season with salt to taste.
4. Serve with whole wheat pita triangles.

Nutrition Information (per serving):

- Calories: 150
- Protein: 5g
- Carbohydrates: 18g
- Fat: 7g
- Fiber: 4g
- Sugar: 1g
- Portion Size: 1/4 cup hummus with whole wheat pita

Greek Yogurt Dip with Cucumber Slices

Ingredients:

- 1 cup Greek yogurt
- 1 teaspoon dill, chopped
- 1 teaspoon lemon zest
- Salt and pepper to taste
- Cucumber, thinly sliced

Instructions:

1. In a bowl, mix Greek yogurt, chopped dill, lemon zest, salt, and pepper.
2. Chill in the refrigerator.
3. Serve with thinly sliced cucumber.

Nutrition Information (per serving):

- Calories: 80
- Protein: 10g
- Carbohydrates: 6g
- Fat: 2g
- Fiber: 1g
- Sugar: 4g

- Portion Size: 1/2 cup yogurt dip with cucumber slices

Roasted Chickpeas

Ingredients:

- 1 can chickpeas, drained and dried
- 1 tablespoon olive oil
- 1 teaspoon paprika
- 1/2 teaspoon cumin
- Salt to taste

Instructions:

1. Preheat oven to 400°F (200°C).
2. Toss chickpeas with olive oil, paprika, cumin, and salt.
3. Spread in a single layer on a baking sheet.
4. Roast for 25-30 minutes, shaking the pan occasionally.
5. Let cool before serving.

Nutrition Information (per serving):

- Calories: 120
- Protein: 5g

- Carbohydrates: 17g

- Fat: 4g

- Fiber: 5g

- Sugar: 3g

- Portion Size: 1/2 cup roasted chickpeas

Sliced Apple with Almond Butter

Ingredients:

- 1 apple, thinly sliced

- 2 tablespoons almond butter

Instructions:

1. Arrange apple slices on a plate.

2. Warm almond butter slightly and drizzle over the apple slices.

Nutrition Information (per serving):

- Calories: 180

- Protein: 3g

- Carbohydrates: 18g

- Fat: 11g

- Fiber: 5g

- Sugar: 12g
- Portion Size: 1 apple with almond butter

Caprese Skewers

Ingredients:

- Cherry tomatoes
- Fresh mozzarella balls
- Fresh basil leaves
- Balsamic glaze for drizzling

Instructions:

1. Thread a cherry tomato, mozzarella ball, and basil leaf onto small skewers.
2. Arrange on a serving platter.
3. Drizzle with balsamic glaze before serving.

Nutrition Information (per serving):

- Calories: 120
- Protein: 7g
- Carbohydrates: 3g
- Fat: 9g
- Fiber: 1g

- Sugar: 1g

- Portion Size: 4 skewers

Edamame with Sea Salt

Ingredients:

- 2 cups edamame, steamed

- Sea salt to taste

Instructions:

1. Steam the edamame according to package instructions.

2. Sprinkle with sea salt before serving.

Nutrition Information (per serving):

- Calories: 150

- Protein: 14g

- Carbohydrates: 11g

- Fat: 6g

- Fiber: 7g

- Sugar: 3g

- Portion Size: 1 cup edamame

Trail Mix with Nuts and Dried Fruits

Ingredients:

- 1/2 cup almonds
- 1/2 cup walnuts
- 1/4 cup dried cranberries
- 1/4 cup raisins
- 1/4 cup dark chocolate chips

Instructions:

1. Mix almonds, walnuts, dried cranberries, raisins, and dark chocolate chips in a bowl.
2. Portion into snack-sized servings.

Nutrition Information (per serving):

- Calories: 200
- Protein: 5g
- Carbohydrates: 18g
- Fat: 14g
- Fiber: 4g
- Sugar: 10g
- Portion Size: 1/2 cup trail mix

Cottage Cheese with Pineapple

Ingredients:

- 1/2 cup low-fat cottage cheese
- 1/2 cup pineapple chunks (fresh or canned)

Instructions:

1. Spoon cottage cheese into a bowl.
2. Top with pineapple chunks.

Nutrition Information (per serving):

- Calories: 120
- Protein: 14g
- Carbohydrates: 15g
- Fat: 1g
- Fiber: 2g
- Sugar: 12g
- Portion Size: 1 cup cottage cheese with pineapple

Stuffed Grape Leaves

Ingredients:

- 1 cup cooked quinoa

- 1/4 cup chopped fresh parsley
- 1 tablespoon lemon juice
- 1 tablespoon olive oil
- Salt and pepper to taste
- Grape leaves (canned or fresh)

Instructions:

1. In a bowl, mix cooked quinoa, chopped parsley, lemon juice, olive oil, salt, and pepper.
2. Spoon the mixture onto grape leaves and roll them up.
3. Serve chilled.

Nutrition Information (per serving):

- Calories: 160
- Protein: 4g
- Carbohydrates: 23g
- Fat: 6g
- Fiber: 3g
- Sugar: 1g
- Portion Size: 4 stuffed grape leaves

Veggie Spring Rolls with Peanut Sauce

Ingredients:

- Rice paper wrappers
- 1 cup julienned carrots
- 1 cup thinly sliced cucumber
- 1 cup sliced bell peppers
- Fresh mint leaves
- 1/4 cup peanut sauce for dipping

Instructions:

1. Dip rice paper wrappers in warm water to soften.
2. Place a small amount of carrots, cucumber, bell peppers, and mint leaves on each wrapper.
3. Roll tightly and serve with peanut sauce.

Nutrition Information (per serving):

- Calories: 180
- Protein: 5g
- Carbohydrates: 30g
- Fat: 5g
- Fiber: 4g

- Sugar: 7g

- Portion Size: 2 spring rolls with peanut sauce

Baked Sweet Potato Fries

Ingredients:

- 2 sweet potatoes, cut into fries

- 1 tablespoon olive oil

- 1 teaspoon paprika

- 1/2 teaspoon garlic powder

- Salt and pepper to taste

Instructions:

1. Preheat oven to 425°F (220°C).

2. Toss sweet potato fries with olive oil, paprika, garlic powder, salt, and pepper.

3. Spread on a baking sheet and bake for 25-30 minutes, flipping halfway through.

Nutrition Information (per serving):

- Calories: 160

- Protein: 2g

- Carbohydrates: 30g

- Fat: 4g
- Fiber: 5g
- Sugar: 6g
- Portion Size: 1 cup baked sweet potato fries

Cheese and Whole Grain Crackers

Ingredients:

- 1 ounce whole grain crackers
- 1 ounce cheese of your choice (cheddar, Swiss, or goat cheese)

Instructions:

1. Arrange whole grain crackers on a plate.
2. Place small slices of cheese on top.

Nutrition Information (per serving):

- Calories: 180
- Protein: 8g
- Carbohydrates: 15g
- Fat: 10g
- Fiber: 3g
- Sugar: 1g

- Portion Size: 1 serving of cheese and crackers

Antipasto Platter with Olives and Cheese

Ingredients:

- Assorted olives (green and black)
- 2 ounces prosciutto
- 2 ounces salami
- 4 ounces mozzarella cheese
- 4 ounces feta cheese
- 1/4 cup marinated artichoke hearts
- 1/4 cup roasted red peppers

Instructions:

1. Arrange olives, prosciutto, salami, mozzarella, feta, artichoke hearts, and roasted red peppers on a platter.

Nutrition Information (per serving):

- Calories: 250
- Protein: 15g
- Carbohydrates: 5g

- Fat: 20g

- Fiber: 2g

- Sugar: 1g

- Portion Size: 1 cup antipasto platter

Cucumber Roll-Ups with Turkey and Cream Cheese

Ingredients:

- 1 large cucumber, thinly sliced lengthwise

- 4 ounces smoked turkey slices

- 4 ounces cream cheese, softened

- Fresh dill for garnish

Instructions:

1. Spread cream cheese over cucumber slices.

2. Place a slice of turkey on each and roll up.

3. Secure with toothpicks and garnish with fresh dill.

Nutrition Information (per serving):

- Calories: 180

- Protein: 10g

- Carbohydrates: 5g

- Fat: 14g

- Fiber: 1g

- Sugar: 3g

- Portion Size: 4 cucumber roll-ups

Chapter 6: Desserts

In this chapter, we present scrumptious dessert recipes that not only satisfy your sweet tooth but also align with prediabetes meal plans. Each recipe is carefully crafted to bring together delicious flavors while considering nutritional aspects. So, let's dive into a realm where taste and health coexist harmoniously.

Berry and Greek Yogurt Popsicles

Ingredients:

- 1 cup mixed berries (strawberries, blueberries, raspberries)
- 1 cup Greek yogurt
- 2 tablespoons honey
- 1 teaspoon vanilla extract

Instructions:

1. In a blender, combine berries, Greek yogurt, honey, and vanilla extract.
2. Blend until smooth.

3. Pour the mixture into popsicle molds.

4. Insert popsicle sticks and freeze for at least 4 hours.

Nutrition Information (per serving):

- Calories: 90
- Protein: 4g
- Carbohydrates: 15g
- Fat: 2g
- Fiber: 2g
- Sugar: 11g
- Portion Size: 1 popsicle

Dark Chocolate-Dipped Strawberries

Ingredients:

- 1 cup dark chocolate chips
- 1 pound fresh strawberries, washed and dried

Instructions:

1. Melt dark chocolate chips in a microwave-safe bowl in 30-second intervals, stirring in between.

2. Dip each strawberry into the melted chocolate, coating them halfway.

3. Place on a parchment paper-lined tray and refrigerate
    until the chocolate sets.

Nutrition Information (per serving):

- Calories: 60
- Protein: 1g
- Carbohydrates: 12g
- Fat: 3g
- Fiber: 3g
- Sugar: 8g
- Portion Size: 4 strawberries

Baked Apples with Cinnamon

Ingredients:

- 4 medium-sized apples, cored and halved
- 2 tablespoons melted butter
- 1 teaspoon cinnamon
- 1 tablespoon honey

Instructions:

1. Preheat the oven to 375°F (190°C).
2. Place apple halves in a baking dish.

3. Mix melted butter, cinnamon, and honey. Brush the
    mixture over the apples.

4. Bake for 25-30 minutes until apples are tender.

Nutrition Information (per serving):

- Calories: 120

- Protein: 1g

- Carbohydrates: 25g

- Fat: 3g

- Fiber: 4g

- Sugar: 18g

- Portion Size: 1 apple half

Almond Flour Banana Bread

Ingredients:

- 2 ripe bananas, mashed

- 3 eggs

- 1/4 cup coconut oil, melted

- 1 teaspoon vanilla extract

- 2 cups almond flour

- 1 teaspoon baking powder

- 1/2 teaspoon cinnamon

Instructions:

1. Preheat the oven to 350°F (175°C).
2. In a bowl, mix mashed bananas, eggs, melted coconut oil, and vanilla extract.
3. Add almond flour, baking powder, and cinnamon. Mix until well combined.
4. Pour the batter into a greased loaf pan and bake for 40-45 minutes.

Nutrition Information (per serving):

- Calories: 180
- Protein: 6g
- Carbohydrates: 10g
- Fat: 14g
- Fiber: 3g
- Sugar: 4g
- Portion Size: 1 slice

Chia Seed Chocolate Pudding

Ingredients:

- 1/4 cup chia seeds
- 1 cup almond milk

- 2 tablespoons cocoa powder
- 1 tablespoon maple syrup
- 1/2 teaspoon vanilla extract

Instructions:

1. Mix chia seeds, almond milk, cocoa powder, maple syrup, and vanilla extract in a bowl.
2. Stir well and refrigerate for at least 2 hours or overnight.
3. Before serving, stir again and top with fresh berries.

Nutrition Information (per serving):

- Calories: 120
- Protein: 4g
- Carbohydrates: 15g
- Fat: 6g
- Fiber: 7g
- Sugar: 4g
- Portion Size: 1/2 cup

Coconut and Berry Parfait

Ingredients:

- 1 cup mixed berries (strawberries, blueberries, raspberries)
- 1 cup coconut yogurt
- 1/4 cup granola
- 2 tablespoons shredded coconut

Instructions:

1. In a glass or bowl, layer coconut yogurt, mixed berries, and granola.
2. Repeat the layers and top with shredded coconut.

Nutrition Information (per serving):

- Calories: 220
- Protein: 5g
- Carbohydrates: 30g
- Fat: 10g
- Fiber: 6g
- Sugar: 15g
- Portion Size: 1 parfait

Mango Sorbet

Ingredients:

- 2 cups frozen mango chunks
- 1/4 cup coconut water
- 1 tablespoon lime juice
- 2 tablespoons honey

Instructions:

1. In a blender, combine frozen mango chunks, coconut water, lime juice, and honey.
2. Blend until smooth and creamy.
3. Transfer the mixture to a shallow dish and freeze for at least 2 hours.

Nutrition Information (per serving):

- Calories: 140
- Protein: 1g
- Carbohydrates: 35g
- Fat: 0.5g
- Fiber: 3g
- Sugar: 30g
- Portion Size: 1/2 cup

Pumpkin Pie Smoothie

Ingredients:

- 1/2 cup canned pumpkin puree
- 1 banana
- 1 cup almond milk
- 1/2 teaspoon pumpkin spice
- 1 tablespoon maple syrup
- Ice cubes (optional)

Instructions:

1. In a blender, combine pumpkin puree, banana, almond milk, pumpkin spice, and maple syrup.
2. Blend until smooth. Add ice cubes if desired.
3. Pour into a glass and sprinkle with a pinch of pumpkin spice.

Nutrition Information (per serving):

- Calories: 160
- Protein: 2g
- Carbohydrates: 35g
- Fat: 2g
- Fiber: 6g

- Sugar: 18g

- Portion Size: 1 smoothie

Oatmeal Raisin Cookies

Ingredients:

- 1 cup old-fashioned oats
- 1/2 cup almond flour
- 1/2 teaspoon cinnamon
- 1/4 teaspoon baking soda
- 1/4 cup coconut oil, melted
- 1/4 cup maple syrup
- 1 teaspoon vanilla extract
- 1/4 cup raisins

Instructions:

1. Preheat the oven to 350°F (175°C) and line a baking sheet with parchment paper.
2. In a bowl, mix oats, almond flour, cinnamon, and baking soda.
3. In a separate bowl, combine melted coconut oil, maple syrup, and vanilla extract.

4. Add the wet ingredients to the dry ingredients and stir until well combined. Fold in raisins.

5. Drop spoonfuls of dough onto the baking sheet and flatten with a fork.

6. Bake for 12-15 minutes or until golden brown.

Nutrition Information (per serving, 2 cookies):

- Calories: 160
- Protein: 3g
- Carbohydrates: 20g
- Fat: 8g
- Fiber: 2g
- Sugar: 9g

Greek Yogurt Cheesecake Bites

Ingredients:

- 1 cup Greek yogurt
- 1/4 cup cream cheese, softened
- 2 tablespoons honey
- 1 teaspoon vanilla extract
- Fresh berries for topping

Instructions:

1. In a bowl, mix Greek yogurt, softened cream cheese, honey, and vanilla extract until smooth.
2. Spoon the mixture into mini muffin cups.
3. Refrigerate for at least 2 hours.
4. Top each with fresh berries before serving.

Nutrition Information (per serving, 2 bites):

- Calories: 120
- Protein: 5g
- Carbohydrates: 10g
- Fat: 6g
- Fiber: 1g
- Sugar: 8g

Lemon Poppy Seed Muffins

Ingredients:

- 2 cups almond flour
- 1/4 cup coconut flour
- 1/2 teaspoon baking soda
- 1/4 teaspoon salt
- 3 eggs

- 1/2 cup coconut oil, melted

- 1/4 cup honey

- Zest and juice of 2 lemons

- 1 tablespoon poppy seeds

Instructions:

1. Preheat the oven to 350°F (175°C) and line a muffin tin with paper liners.

2. In a bowl, whisk together almond flour, coconut flour, baking soda, and salt.

3. In another bowl, beat eggs, melted coconut oil, honey, lemon zest, and lemon juice.

4. Add wet ingredients to dry and mix until combined. Fold in poppy seeds.

5. Spoon the batter into the muffin cups and bake for 18-20 minutes.

Nutrition Information (per serving, 1 muffin):

- Calories: 180

- Protein: 5g

- Carbohydrates: 10g

- Fat: 14g

- Fiber: 3g

- Sugar: 5g

Mixed Berry Crisp

Ingredients:

- 3 cups mixed berries (strawberries, blueberries, raspberries)
- 1 tablespoon lemon juice
- 1/4 cup maple syrup
- 1 cup rolled oats
- 1/2 cup almond flour
- 1/4 cup coconut oil, melted
- 1/4 cup chopped nuts (optional)

Instructions:

1. Preheat the oven to 350°F (175°C).
2. In a bowl, toss mixed berries with lemon juice and maple syrup. Transfer to a baking dish.
3. In another bowl, mix rolled oats, almond flour, melted coconut oil, and nuts.
4. Sprinkle the oat mixture over the berries.

5. Bake for 25-30 minutes or until the topping is golden brown.

Nutrition Information (per serving):

- Calories: 220
- Protein: 4g
- Carbohydrates: 30g
- Fat: 10g
- Fiber: 6g
- Sugar: 15g
- Portion Size: 1/2 cup

Avocado Chocolate Mousse

Ingredients:

- 2 ripe avocados
- 1/4 cup cocoa powder
- 1/4 cup almond milk
- 1/4 cup maple syrup
- 1 teaspoon vanilla extract
- Pinch of salt

Instructions:

1. Scoop out the avocados and place them in a blender.

2. Add cocoa powder, almond milk, maple syrup, vanilla extract, and a pinch of salt.

3. Blend until smooth and creamy.

4. Refrigerate for at least 1 hour before serving.

Nutrition Information (per serving):

*   Calories: 160

*   Protein: 3g

*   Carbohydrates: 15g

*   Fat: 11g

*   Fiber: 6g

*   Sugar: 6g

*   Portion Size: 1/2 cup

Peach and Almond Crumble

Ingredients:

*   4 cups sliced peaches

*   1 tablespoon lemon juice

*   2 tablespoons maple syrup

*   1/2 teaspoon almond extract

- 1 cup almond flour
- 1/2 cup rolled oats
- 1/4 cup coconut oil, melted
- 2 tablespoons sliced almonds

Instructions:

1. Preheat the oven to 350°F (175°C).
2. In a bowl, combine sliced peaches, lemon juice, maple syrup, and almond extract. Transfer to a baking dish.
3. In another bowl, mix almond flour, rolled oats, melted coconut oil, and sliced almonds.
4. Sprinkle the almond mixture over the peaches.
5. Bake for 30-35 minutes or until the topping is golden brown.

Nutrition Information (per serving):

- Calories: 230
- Protein: 5g
- Carbohydrates: 25g
- Fat: 14g
- Fiber: 5g

- Sugar: 15g
- Portion Size: 1/2 cup

Raspberry and Almond Energy Bites

Ingredients:

- 1 cup almonds
- 1 cup dried raspberries
- 1/4 cup chia seeds
- 2 tablespoons coconut oil, melted
- 1/4 cup honey
- 1 teaspoon almond extract
- Shredded coconut for rolling

Instructions:

1. In a food processor, combine almonds, dried raspberries, and chia seeds. Pulse until finely ground.
2. Add melted coconut oil, honey, and almond extract. Blend until the mixture comes together.
3. Roll the mixture into bite-sized balls and coat with shredded coconut.
4. Refrigerate for at least 1 hour before serving.

Nutrition Information (per serving, 2 bites):

- Calories: 140
- Protein: 4g
- Carbohydrates: 14g
- Fat: 8g
- Fiber: 4g
- Sugar: 8g

Chapter 7: Smoothies

These delightful concoctions not only promise a burst of deliciousness but also pack a punch of nutritional goodness. Dive into a world of refreshing ingredients and invigorating blends that will make healthy living a delicious endeavor. Each smoothie is carefully curated to bring you a unique experience, ensuring you stay on track with your prediabetes meal plan.

Green Detox Smoothie

Ingredients:

- 1 cup fresh spinach leaves
- 1/2 cucumber, peeled and sliced
- 1 green apple, cored and chopped
- 1/2 lemon, juiced
- 1 cup coconut water
- Ice cubes (optional)

Instructions:

1. Combine spinach, cucumber, apple, lemon juice, and coconut water in a blender.
2. Blend until smooth.
3. Add ice cubes if desired and blend again.
4. Pour into a glass and enjoy!

Nutrition Information:

- Calories: 120
- Protein: 3g
- Carbohydrates: 28g
- Fat: 1g
- Fiber: 5g
- Sugar: 18g
- Portion Size: 1 serving

Berry Blast Smoothie

Ingredients:

- 1 cup mixed berries (strawberries, blueberries, raspberries)
- 1/2 banana
- 1/2 cup Greek yogurt

- 1 tablespoon chia seeds

- 1 cup almond milk

- Ice cubes (optional)

Instructions:

1. Combine mixed berries, banana, Greek yogurt, chia seeds, and almond milk in a blender.
2. Blend until smooth.
3. Add ice cubes if desired and blend again.
4. Pour into a glass and savor the berry goodness!

Nutrition Information:

- Calories: 180

- Protein: 7g

- Carbohydrates: 25g

- Fat: 6g

- Fiber: 8g

- Sugar: 13g

- Portion Size: 1 serving

Tropical Paradise Smoothie

Ingredients:

- 1/2 cup pineapple chunks
- 1/2 cup mango chunks
- 1/2 banana
- 1/2 cup coconut milk
- 1 tablespoon flaxseeds
- Ice cubes (optional)

Instructions:

1. Combine pineapple, mango, banana, coconut milk, and flaxseeds in a blender.
2. Blend until smooth.
3. Add ice cubes if desired and blend again.
4. Pour into a glass and transport yourself to a tropical paradise!

Nutrition Information:

- Calories: 200
- Protein: 5g
- Carbohydrates: 30g
- Fat: 8g

- Fiber: 6g

- Sugar: 18g

- Portion Size: 1 serving

Avocado and Spinach Smoothie

Ingredients:

- 1/2 avocado, peeled and pitted

- 1 cup fresh spinach leaves

- 1/2 cup cucumber, sliced

- 1/2 lime, juiced

- 1 cup almond milk

- Ice cubes (optional)

Instructions:

1. Combine avocado, spinach, cucumber, lime juice, and almond milk in a blender.

2. Blend until creamy and smooth.

3. Add ice cubes if desired and blend again.

4. Pour into a glass and relish the creamy texture.

Nutrition Information:

- Calories: 160

- Protein: 5g

- Carbohydrates: 12g

- Fat: 11g

- Fiber: 7g

- Sugar: 2g

- Portion Size: 1 serving

Almond Butter Banana Smoothie

Ingredients:

- 1 banana

- 2 tablespoons almond butter

- 1/2 cup Greek yogurt

- 1 cup almond milk

- 1 tablespoon honey

- Ice cubes (optional)

Instructions:

1. Combine banana, almond butter, Greek yogurt, almond milk, and honey in a blender.

2. Blend until silky smooth.

3. Add ice cubes if desired and blend again.

4. Pour into a glass and relish the nutty sweetness.

Nutrition Information:

- Calories: 250
- Protein: 9g
- Carbohydrates: 30g
- Fat: 12g
- Fiber: 5g
- Sugar: 18g
- Portion Size: 1 serving

Blueberry and Kale Smoothie

Ingredients:

- 1/2 cup blueberries
- 1 cup kale leaves, stems removed
- 1/2 banana
- 1/2 cup plain yogurt
- 1 tablespoon flaxseeds
- 1 cup water
- Ice cubes (optional)

Instructions:

1. Combine blueberries, kale, banana, yogurt, flaxseeds, and water in a blender.

2. Blend until vibrant and smooth.

3. Add ice cubes if desired and blend again.

4. Pour into a glass and enjoy the antioxidant-rich blend.

Nutrition Information:

- Calories: 140
- Protein: 6g
- Carbohydrates: 25g
- Fat: 4g
- Fiber: 8g
- Sugar: 12g
- Portion Size: 1 serving

Pineapple Mint Smoothie

Ingredients:

- 1 cup pineapple chunks
- Handful of fresh mint leaves
- 1/2 lime, juiced
- 1/2 banana
- 1/2 cup coconut water
- Ice cubes (optional)

Instructions:

1. Combine pineapple, mint leaves, lime juice, banana, and coconut water in a blender.
2. Blend until the mint is finely incorporated, and the mixture is smooth.
3. Add ice cubes if desired and blend again.
4. Pour into a glass and savor the tropical freshness.

Nutrition Information:

- Calories: 160
- Protein: 3g
- Carbohydrates: 38g
- Fat: 1g
- Fiber: 5g
- Sugar: 22g
- Portion Size: 1 serving

Cucumber and Mint Smoothie

Ingredients:

- 1/2 cucumber, peeled and sliced
- Handful of fresh mint leaves
- 1/2 green apple, cored and chopped

- 1/2 lemon, juiced

- 1 cup water

- Ice cubes (optional)

Instructions:

1. Combine cucumber, mint leaves, green apple, lemon juice, and water in a blender.
2. Blend until the mixture is smooth and refreshing.
3. Add ice cubes if desired and blend again.
4. Pour into a glass and enjoy the hydrating goodness.

Nutrition Information:

- Calories: 80

- Protein: 2g

- Carbohydrates: 20g

- Fat: 0.5g

- Fiber: 4g

- Sugar: 12g

- Portion Size: 1 serving

Chocolate Avocado Smoothie

Ingredients:

- 1/2 avocado, peeled and pitted
- 1 tablespoon cocoa powder
- 1/2 banana
- 1 cup almond milk
- 1 tablespoon honey
- Ice cubes (optional)

Instructions:

1. Combine avocado, cocoa powder, banana, almond milk, and honey in a blender.
2. Blend until the mixture is rich and chocolatey.
3. Add ice cubes if desired and blend again.
4. Pour into a glass and indulge in the guilt-free chocolate treat.

Nutrition Information:

- Calories: 220
- Protein: 5g
- Carbohydrates: 25g
- Fat: 14g

- Fiber: 7g
- Sugar: 13g
- Portion Size: 1 serving

Mango Tango Smoothie

Ingredients:

- 1 cup mango chunks
- 1/2 cup pineapple chunks
- 1/2 banana
- 1/2 cup Greek yogurt
- 1 tablespoon chia seeds
- 1 cup coconut water
- Ice cubes (optional)

Instructions:

1. Combine mango, pineapple, banana, Greek yogurt, chia seeds, and coconut water in a blender.
2. Blend until the mixture is smooth and tropical.
3. Add ice cubes if desired and blend again.
4. Pour into a glass and dance your taste buds through the mango tango.

Nutrition Information:

- Calories: 190
- Protein: 7g
- Carbohydrates: 30g
- Fat: 6g
- Fiber: 8g
- Sugar: 20g
- Portion Size: 1 serving

Orange Creamsicle Smoothie

Ingredients:

- 1 orange, peeled and segmented
- 1/2 banana
- 1/2 cup Greek yogurt
- 1/2 cup almond milk
- 1 tablespoon flaxseeds
- Ice cubes (optional)

Instructions:

1. Combine orange segments, banana, Greek yogurt, almond milk, and flaxseeds in a blender.

2. Blend until the mixture is creamy and reminiscent of a creamsicle.

3. Add ice cubes if desired and blend again.

4. Pour into a glass and relish the citrusy sweetness.

Nutrition Information:

- Calories: 160
- Protein: 6g
- Carbohydrates: 25g
- Fat: 5g
- Fiber: 7g
- Sugar: 15g
- Portion Size: 1 serving

Pomegranate and Raspberry Smoothie

Ingredients:

- 1/2 cup pomegranate seeds
- 1/2 cup raspberries
- 1/2 banana
- 1/2 cup plain yogurt

- 1 cup water
- Ice cubes (optional)

Instructions:

1. Combine pomegranate seeds, raspberries, banana, yogurt, and water in a blender.
2. Blend until the mixture is vibrant and luscious.
3. Add ice cubes if desired and blend again.
4. Pour into a glass and savor the antioxidant-packed goodness.

Nutrition Information:

- Calories: 140
- Protein: 4g
- Carbohydrates: 30g
- Fat: 1g
- Fiber: 8g
- Sugar: 18g
- Portion Size: 1 serving

Spinach and Pineapple Smoothie

Ingredients:

- 1 cup fresh spinach leaves
- 1/2 cup pineapple chunks
- 1/2 banana
- 1/2 cup coconut water
- 1 tablespoon chia seeds
- Ice cubes (optional)

Instructions:

1. Combine spinach, pineapple, banana, coconut water, and chia seeds in a blender.
2. Blend until the mixture is smooth and nutrient-packed.
3. Add ice cubes if desired and blend again.
4. Pour into a glass and enjoy the green goodness.

Nutrition Information:

- Calories: 120
- Protein: 4g
- Carbohydrates: 25g
- Fat: 3g

- Fiber: 6g
- Sugar: 15g
- Portion Size: 1 serving

Coffee and Almond Milk Smoothie

Ingredients:
- 1/2 cup brewed coffee, cooled
- 1/2 banana
- 1 tablespoon almond butter
- 1 cup almond milk
- 1 tablespoon honey
- Ice cubes (optional)

Instructions:
1. Combine brewed coffee, banana, almond butter, almond milk, and honey in a blender.
2. Blend until the mixture is velvety and caffeinated.
3. Add ice cubes if desired and blend again.
4. Pour into a glass and revel in the coffee-infused delight.

Nutrition Information:

- Calories: 180
- Protein: 5g
- Carbohydrates: 20g
- Fat: 10g
- Fiber: 4g
- Sugar: 12g
- Portion Size: 1 serving

Carrot Cake Smoothie

Ingredients:

- 1/2 cup shredded carrots
- 1/2 banana
- 1/4 cup rolled oats
- 1/2 teaspoon cinnamon
- 1 cup almond milk
- 1 tablespoon maple syrup
- Ice cubes (optional)

Instructions:

1. Combine shredded carrots, banana, rolled oats, cinnamon, almond milk, and maple syrup in a blender.
2. Blend until the mixture is reminiscent of carrot cake goodness.
3. Add ice cubes if desired and blend again.
4. Pour into a glass and savor the dessert-like experience.

Nutrition Information:

- Calories: 170
- Protein: 4g
- Carbohydrates: 30g
- Fat: 4g
- Fiber: 5g
- Sugar: 14g
- Portion Size: 1 serving

CONCLUSION

In concluding this Prediabetes Cookbooks Meal Plans guide, we embark on a collective celebration of newfound knowledge and nourishment. Throughout these pages, we've explored the intricate symphony of flavors, textures, and nutritional values designed to empower individuals on their journey toward better health.

Our 30-day meal plan serves not only as a roadmap but as a testament to the delightful possibilities that lie within every mindful bite. From invigorating breakfasts that kickstart your day to satisfying dinners that bring closure to your culinary exploration, each recipe has been carefully crafted with the principles of balanced and prediabetes-friendly nutrition.

As we close this chapter, it's crucial to recognize that this isn't just a cookbook—it's a companion on your path to wellness. The recipes provided are more than just a list of ingredients; they represent a commitment to embracing a lifestyle that promotes well-being and nourishes both body and soul.

Remember, this journey doesn't end here. The true success of this guide lies in the continued incorporation of these mindful eating habits into your daily life. Whether you're savoring a nutrient-packed smoothie, relishing a wholesome dinner, or enjoying a guilt-free dessert, each choice is a step toward a healthier, more vibrant you.

As you savor the flavors and experience the positive changes in your well-being, take pride in the commitment you've made to your health. With knowledge, determination, and these delicious recipes in hand, you are well-equipped to navigate the path ahead—one that leads to sustained vitality and a fulfilling life.

May your culinary adventures continue to be as rewarding as they are delicious, and may this cookbook be a constant source of inspiration and guidance on your ongoing journey toward a healthier, happier you. Cheers to a life well-lived, full of vibrant health and the joy that comes from nourishing your body with love and intention.

www.ingramcontent.com/pod-product-compliance
Lightning Source LLC
Chambersburg PA
CBHW070949260726
48661CB00003B/1200